# OBESITY

# OBESITY

**by Daniel McMillan**

A Venture Book
**Franklin Watts**
New York  Chicago  London  Toronto  Sydney

Library of Congress Cataloging-in-Publication Data

McMillan, Daniel.
Obesity / by Daniel McMillan.
p.     cm. — (A Venture book)
Includes bibliographical references and index.
ISBN 0-531-11201-2 (lib. bdg.)
1. Obesity—Juvenile literature.   [1. Obesity.   2. Weight
control.]   I. Title.
RC628.M38   1994
616.3'98—dc20                            94-21033   CIP   AC

# CONTENTS

# OBESITY

# INTRODUCTION

*Has it ever struck you that there's a thin man inside every fat man, just as they say there's a statue inside every block of stone?*

George Orwell,
*Coming Up for Air*, 1939

An estimated 30 million Americans—a little more than 10 percent of the U.S. population—are obese. Public health specialists consider obesity this nation's most serious nutritional problem; it is a leading risk factor for many of the deadliest (and costliest) human health conditions, including cardiovascular disease, cancer, and diabetes. Treatment of obesity, while greatly advanced by recent behavioral, surgical, and pharmacological developments, remains disappointing. Only about 10 percent of obese individuals achieve permanent reversal of their condition.[1]

Such facts detail a less than optimistic scenario, but obese persons also suffer additional burdens. While health professionals recognize obesity as a serious health concern, in a number of important respects obesity is viewed differently than other common human health disorders. For one thing, serious social stigmas are associated with obesity. In contrast to people who suffer from many other health problems, the obese are commonly blamed for their own condition, and reviled as lazy, weak-willed people who do not make the effort to take care of their physical health. As Dr. George Bray, a leading obesity specialist, has pointed out, "the public perceives obesity not as a 'disease' . . . but rather as the result of gluttony and a lack of willpower. Most people believe that the power to push oneself away from the table is all that is needed to treat obesity."[2]

In some cases, the stigma of obesity goes beyond simple misconceptions about how the disorder develops. It is not unusual for normal-weight persons to feel outright revulsion for obese individuals' bodily dimensions. Obese people are all too well aware of the contempt many others feel toward them and they frequently react, justifiably, with anger and withdrawal.

Obesity also differs from other health conditions because, in addition to serious physical difficulties—life-threatening cardiovascular disease, painful arthritis caused by increased strain on weight-bearing joints, everyday discomforts such as that occasioned by sitting in an average-sized movie theater seat —it also involves great psychological burdens. Feelings of social isolation and of depression over the inability to control body weight are widespread in the obese population. The severe ridicule many obese individuals face throughout their lives, particularly during childhood and adolescence, can have lifelong consequences.

These are just some of the factors that differentiate obesity from other common health problems. An examination of obesity must therefore address these elements.

Conversely, an exploration of obesity also parallels studies of other major health problems people face today. For example, like cancer, obesity is the subject of a great deal of medical research through which doctors and other health professionals are attempting to uncover clues about the disease, how it develops, and how it can be treated. As with many other chronic health problems, obesity is a complex disorder with roots that extend in many different directions, including genetics, lifestyles, and environmental surroundings. The study of obesity is particularly fascinating because, although it is a very common condition, so much about it remains to be understood. In the meantime, there is considerable controversy regarding some key aspects of this disorder. This book will attempt to illuminate some of these controversies.

In this book, obesity will be examined as a human health issue with special emphasis placed on medical aspects of this disorder. Psychological and social considerations will also be addressed. The ultimate aim is to contribute to a broad-based understanding of obesity in the hope that readers will recognize that this is a widespread and serious health condition and that individuals who suffer from it require compassion and support rather than derision and disdain.

Writing this book required the assistance of many people and organizations. The University of Iowa library system was invaluable in supplying resources, as were several friends who provided useful documents and important personal perspectives.

# 1
# A THIN
# PERSON'S WORLD

*Persons who desire to become plump and remain so should
retire about 9 or 10 P.M., and sleep until 6 or 7 A.M. A brain-
worker needs more sleep than a muscle-worker.*

*The breakfast should be plain and substantial, the year
round, especially in summer. A course of fresh ripe fruit
should first be eaten, then potatoes, meat or fried mush, or
oat-meal porridge, bread and butter. The drink may be cocoa
or milk-and-water, sweetened.*

*The hearty meal of the day should not come later than
five hours after breakfast. About 3 or 4 P.M., a drink of water
should be taken. Supper should be light; bread-and-butter
and tea, with some mild sauce. Children and old people should
retire early.*

*Another method of becoming plump is a free diet of
oysters. They may be taken in any form, raw or cooked, but
they should be eaten without vinegar or pepper. To sum up,
then: to become plump, one must use plenty of water, starchy
food, oysters, fats, vegetables, sweets, and take plenty of rest.*

In their 1901 book *Vitalogy or Encyclopedia of Health and
Home* physicians George P. Wood and E. H. Ruddock
devoted a section called "How to Become Fat or
Plump" especially to fattening techniques. "This is

more easily accomplished than is generally supposed," wrote the authors, as if they had to convince their readers. "By following the instructions," they promised the doubtful, "lean or spare persons will become fleshy or plump."

Modern readers can find humor in the course of action proposed by the good Drs. Wood and Ruddock. First of all, medical professionals today would be loath to recommend a regimen specifically designed to fatten an otherwise healthy patient. To be sure, the prescription offered by Wood and Ruddock merely reflects the prevailing wisdom of their day, which equated "plumpness" with robust health. That notion has fallen out of favor as medical science has discovered the many health hazards associated with excess weight.

Secondly, aside from health concerns, fewer and fewer people today actually "desire to become plump and remain so" for aesthetic purposes. Like so many other things, views on physical attractiveness have changed dramatically since the days of the early twentieth century. Conceptions of physical beauty are transitory at best.

Despite the fact that definitions of beauty are ever-changing, the amount of time, money, and effort many people spend in search of this elusive ideal is truly remarkable. In 1990, the Federal Trade Commission estimated that Americans spent $30 billion in the effort to lose weight.[1] According to some estimates, cosmetics companies earned $50 million in 1992 just through the sale of "anti-cellulite" creams, lotions purported to eliminate unsightly fat ripples. Never mind that most doctors and the Federal Trade Commission dispute the efficacy of such creams.

In the United States and most other developed countries today, the extraordinary emphasis placed on physical attractiveness and the preoccupation with beauty is coupled with extreme pressure to conform to a standard anatomic shape if one is to qualify as "desirable." Specifically, for both males and females, the slender, muscular physique is now considered to be the primary component of physical attractiveness.

Cultural forces perpetuate such notions of the desirable body type while simultaneously devaluing other physiques, particularly the overweight or obese. Film and television celebrities, with very few exceptions, are gifted with wondrous physical attributes, if not with acting ability; professional and amateur athletes, strong and well conditioned, are among our most admired public figures; new clothing styles are unveiled only on the most slender fashion models; even popular children's dolls are endowed with fashion model figures. The result is a collective impression that slim body types are preferable, and well worth possessing at any price.

Living in such a world, individuals who fail to conform to these standards often find themselves dismissed, ignored, or even scorned and mistreated. Those whose body shape is furthest from the prescribed beauty ideal—obese individuals—face tremendous barriers, including prejudice, discrimination, and psychological abuse.*

---

* While the unfair treatment of those who do not conform to prevailing notions of beauty is certainly unjust, the importance of physical fitness must not be dismissed. It is well known that physical fitness, particularly healthy body weight, is an important component in overall health; conversely, excess body weight is associated with multiple adverse health effects. The purpose of the above discussion is simply to point out that our society, through its many reinforcing mechanisms, has elevated a very specific body type—the slim, muscular build—to a place of great honor and, in doing so, has created very real pressures on people to fashion themselves accordingly. Those who do not or cannot emulate the standard are frequently penalized.

The hurt inflicted on these people can be crippling. Some studies indicate that the obese are less likely to be hired or promoted than normal-weight people with the same qualifications. There is also some evidence that obesity negatively affects one's chances of being accepted to top-notch educational institutions.[2] The case of Sharon Russell, a 300-pound nursing student who claimed she was expelled from a Rhode Island college in 1985 because of her excess weight, drew national attention to a form of discrimination often overlooked or denied.

Before leaving the topic of attitudes toward attractiveness and desirability, and for the sake of further perspective on this issue, it is worth noting that different cultures value different physical attributes. In fact, many cultures would likely consider the average New York fashion model severely undernourished. Everyone who has seen a *National Geographic* magazine can testify to the latitude that is allowed in applying the term "beautiful."

Even within a given culture, perceptions of what is and is not a desirable body type are constantly changing over time, as the quote from Wood and Ruddock indicates. The paintings of artists such as Peter Paul Rubens (1577–1640), François Boucher (1703–70), and Pierre-Auguste Renoir (1841–1919) provide additional evidence of this fact. The nudes they depict are overweight by today's standard, yet they represented the physical ideal of their day.

Qualities such as beauty and desirability are given new meaning by every age and culture. By recognizing that definitions of attractiveness are ever shifting, it is possible to appreciate individuals who do not fit into these narrow categories. After all, such individuals constitute the *majority* of our population. This book will focus on one specific group of people, the obese, who do not conform to our culture's standard definition of beautiful.

## DEFINING OBESITY

In general terms, obesity is characterized by the accumulation of an excessive amount of fatty or adipose tissue. The presence of this excess fat impairs the functioning of many important organs and body systems and can lead to multiple other health problems, even death. Technically, obesity is distinct from overweight, which is an accumulation of excess *body weight* (not necessarily fat), although the two terms are often used interchangeably.

Defining obesity has proven to be difficult for health professionals concerned with this disorder. The National Institutes of Health has described obesity as "an excess of body fat frequently resulting in a significant impairment of health." But the point at which an impairment of health is seen cannot always be determined very precisely. The United States Public Health Service publication *Healthy People 2000*—the so-called blueprint for the nation's health—acknowledges the absence of a standard definition: "An ideal, health-oriented definition of obesity would be based on the degree of excess body fat at which health risks to individuals begin to increase. No such definition exists."

Given the lack of uniformity in defining the problem, most doctors rely upon their powers of observation (the so-called eyeball test), at least initially, to arrive at a diagnosis of obesity. As bluntly stated by childhood obesity specialist Dr. Leonard Taitz: "Someone is obese when they look obese."[3]

This rather imprecise definition of obesity has not prevented researchers from developing several useful classification systems for obesity (these will be discussed later in this chapter). These classification systems have helped health professionals to investigate this disorder in its many variations and to specify links between excess body fat and a long list of adverse health consequences, including cardiovascular disease, diabetes, high blood pressure, cancer, arthritis, gallbladder disease, and certain reproductive disorders. Yet a great many questions remain, not the least of which is where to draw the line dividing people of "normal" body weight, or even "acceptable plumpness," from those considered obese.

## SCOPE OF THE PROBLEM

The vast majority of experts acknowledge that obesity, however it is defined, is prevalent enough to be considered a serious public health concern in North America. It is estimated that approximately 10 to 12 percent of adults in the United States (about 30 million people) are obese. The 1988 Surgeon General's Report on Nutrition and Health ranks obesity as the top nutritional problem in the United States. Worldwide, obesity is also a significant problem, particularly in affluent countries.

Ironically, these high levels of obesity exist within a culture that very nearly worships the thin body. Even though at any one time 25 percent of men and 50 percent of women in the United States claim to be dieting to lose weight, the incidence of obesity continues to climb, according to a study.[4] The cost of obesity is also staggering. One researcher investigating the economic costs of obesity, including expenses resulting from chronic conditions brought on by obesity, concluded that "the sum of the costs attributable to obesity . . . is $39.3 billion, which represents 5.5% of total cost of illness in 1986."[5]

Thus, even though there is not a universally accepted definition of obesity, there is a consensus that the condition causes serious health problems, costs the nation a great deal of money, and should be treated.

The *Healthy People 2000* report emphasizes the adoption of habits that allow individuals to "attain an appropriate body weight." Specifically, the report calls for concerted public health efforts to increase to at least 50 percent the proportion of overweight people aged twelve and older who have adopted sound dietary practices combined with regular physical activity. (The National Health Interview Survey conducted in 1985 by the U.S. Centers for Disease Control found that only 30 percent of overweight women and only 25 percent of overweight men aged eighteen and older were attempting to control their body weight.) The Public Health Service's report states:

> *. . . Given the potential health benefits of weight loss in the overweight person, this objective deserves special priority. Attaining this objective will help to reduce the prevalence of overweight in the total population. The prevention of overweight among those not yet overweight is also vitally important.*[6]

## IDENTIFYING OBESITY

Despite the absence of an "ideal" definition of obesity, it is still necessary for health professionals to gather information about overfat patients and to appropriately diagnose and treat this condition. In addition to the "eyeball test," sophisticated techniques and formulas are regularly employed to gauge body composition and thereby diagnose obesity.

One common benchmark is the determination of body fat content. In adult males, obesity has been defined as body fat content greater than 25 percent of total body weight. In adult females, fat content greater than 30 percent of total body weight is often considered obese. In "normal" eighteen-year-old males, about 15 to 18 percent of total body weight is fat, while the corresponding figure for "normal" females is 20 to 25 percent. These percentages vary with age. Infants usually possess about 12 percent body fat at birth; by age six months, the percentage jumps to approximately 25. Through adolescence, fat content slips to around 15 percent of total body weight. At puberty, however, most females can expect to experience significant increases in fat accumulation, usually to about 20 to 25 percent, while fat content in pubescent males remains mostly stable or declines somewhat. With increasing age, fat percentages generally rise in both men and women, reaching 30 to 40 percent of body weight in many cases.

A number of methods are used to gauge body fat percentages, none of which are absolutely reliable. Measurements of skin-fold thickness, in which a trained technician uses a device called a caliper to gently pinch sections of skin at selected body locations, can yield an estimate of body fat percentage. Certain weighing techniques, including underwater weighing, may also be employed. New technology, including devices which measure the movement of electrical impulses through body tissue, may provide highly accurate estimates of body fat, but such equipment is not usually available in the average medical office.

Estimates of body fat content are derived from an individual's weight and height. These estimations are probably the most popular measures in use today because of the ease of collecting weight and height data. One of the primary weight/height-based measures is called Body Mass Index (BMI), which has been shown to correlate quite closely with body fat. The BMI figure is usually arrived at by dividing a person's bodily weight in kilograms by the square of his or her height in meters ($W \div H^2 = BMI$). For instance, someone weighing 75 kilograms (about 165 pounds) and standing 1.8 meters (about 5 feet, 10 inches) would have a 23.1 BMI. (See Table 1–1 for metric conversions of weight and height. See Table 1–2 for information on determining BMI.)

Target BMI figures for males and females in various age groups have been established by the National Institutes of Health, some life insurance companies, and independent researchers. (See Table 1–3.) Using such BMI targets, obesity may be defined as a BMI greater than 30. As BMI increases, so does the level of risk for health problems such as cardiovascular and gallbladder disease, and diabetes. Research has shown that people with a BMI of 20 to 25 have the lowest death rates. In contrast, individuals with a BMI in excess of 40 have death rates three times greater than those of people with a BMI of 20.

**TABLE 1-1.** *Metric Conversions for Weight and Height*
*(2.2 pounds = 1 kilogram)*
*(39.4 inches = 1 meter)*

| WEIGHT | | HEIGHT | |
|---|---|---|---|
| Pounds | Kilograms | Inches | Meters |
| 110 | 50 | 60 | 1.52 |
| 130 | 59 | 62 | 1.57 |
| 150 | 68 | 64 | 1.63 |
| 170 | 77 | 66 | 1.68 |
| 190 | 86 | 68 | 1.73 |
| 210 | 95 | 70 | 1.78 |
| 230 | 105 | 72 | 1.83 |
| 250 | 114 | 74 | 1.88 |

## TABLE 1-2. *Determining BMI*
### *Nomogram for Body Mass Index*

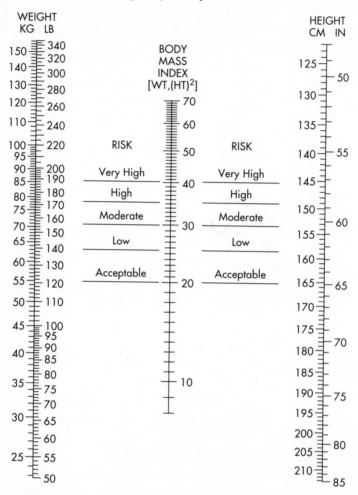

To use this chart, place a ruler or other straightedge between the column on the left (weight) and the column on the right (height). The point where the straightedge crosses the middle scale shows BMI.

**TABLE 1-3.** *Desirable Body Mass Index Range According to Age*

| Age in years | Body Mass Index (kg/m²) |
|:---:|:---:|
| 19-24 | 19-24 |
| 25-34 | 20-25 |
| 35-44 | 21-26 |
| 45-54 | 22-27 |
| 55-64 | 23-28 |
| 65+ | 24-29 |

Source: Bray, G.A.: *The Obese Patient. Major Problems in Internal Medicine.* W.B. Saunders, Philadelphia, 1976.

## CLASSIFICATION SYSTEMS

A number of systems of classification have been developed by researchers investigating obesity. Various systems are based on

- the severity of the disorder
- the anatomic characteristics and distribution of body fat
- the age at which obesity developed
- the factors that contributed to the onset of obesity

Because obesity is a complex condition, originating from multiple sources and associated with serious health consequences, classification is an important first step in determining appropriate treatments.

## SEVERITY OF THE DISORDER

Classifications systems based on the severity of obesity are common. Table 1–4 shows a system developed on the basis of degree of overweight using BMI data. This kind of classification results in familiar categories like overweight, obese, morbidly obese, and super obese. Other classification systems based on degree of overweight determine a person's percentage above ideal body weight. (Two commonly used cut-off points to determine obesity are 120 percent of ideal body weight and 135 percent of ideal body weight.)

Still other classification systems take into account the severity of coexisting medical problems such as high blood pressure, degenerative arthritis, diabetes, or respiratory disease. In addition, it is possible to classify

**TABLE 1-4.** *Classes of Obesity by Degree of Overweight*

|  | MEN | | WOMEN | |
|---|---|---|---|---|
|  | % of IBW | BMI | % of IBW | BMI |
| Ideal Body Weight | 100 | 22 | 100 | 21 |
| Overweight | 110 | 25 | 120 | 25 |
| Obese | 135 | 30 | 145 | 30 |
| Medically Significant Obesity | 160 | 35 | 170 | 35 |
| Morbid Obesity | 200 | 45 | 220 | 45 |
| Super Obesity | 225 | >50 | 245 | >50 |
| IBW = Ideal Body Weight | | | | |

Source: Forse, A, Benott, PN, Blackburn, GL: "Morbid obesity: Weighing the treatment options–surgical intervention." *Nutrition Today*, Sept./Oct. 1989.

the severity of obesity on the basis of age or the speed at which excessive weight is accumulating.

## ANATOMIC CHARACTERISTICS
## AND FAT DISTRIBUTION

The anatomic characteristics of fatty (or adipose) tissue includes both the number and size of fat cells and the distribution of fat throughout the body. Sometimes doctors estimate the number and size of fat cells in a person's body by collecting a sample of adipose tissue. More frequently, body fat is estimated through observation and the determination of the onset of obesity.

The regional distribution of fat on the body can be easily determined using instruments available in most doctors' offices. Measuring skin folds with calipers at several sites on the body is one of the easiest and most widely used techniques. Determination of the waist-hips ratio (ratio of the circumference of the waist to that of the hips) is another common indicator of fat distribution. Some doctors believe the waist-hips ratio is particularly valuable, not only because it can be more reliably measured than skin folds, but also because large ratios may accurately predict the onset of certain obesity-related diseases. In general, men are more likely to have high waist-hip ratios, because they usually have more upper body fat than women.

It is important to identify the regional distribution of excess body fat for several reasons. First, certain health effects can be predicted by determining the primary location of fat deposition. A person with fat located mainly in the abdominal area may be at greater risk of hypertension, heart disease, and diabetes mellitus than a person with more adipose tissue mainly in the buttocks and thighs.

Secondly, classifying obesity according to regional

distribution also provides hints about metabolic characteristics of the individual. For instance, someone with excessive fat accumulation around the thighs, hips, and buttocks (so-called gynecoid or female-type obesity) is less likely to suffer metabolic complications than an individual with obesity localized in the abdominal region. Such information can be useful in the treatment of obesity.

Table 1–5 describes one system for classifying obesity according to the pattern of excess fat distribution.

**TABLE 1-5.** *Types of Obesity by Anatomical Distribution of Body Fat*

| Type I | Excess BMI or fat percentage; no particular concentration in any one area |
|---|---|
| Type II | Excess subcutaneous fat on the trunk, particularly the abdominal region (also called android or male type obesity) |
| Type III | Excess fat in the abdominal visceral area |
| Type IV | Excess fat in the buttocks and thighs (also called gynoid or female type obesity) |

Source: Bouchard, C., "Current understanding of the etiology of obesity: Genetic and nongenetic factors." *American Journal of Clinical Nutrition*, 53:1561S, 1991.

## AGE

Obesity can occur at any age from infancy to late adulthood, although most obesity develops between age 6 and age 20.[7] With few exceptions, childhood obesity is not necessarily an indicator of obesity in adulthood. In the case of women, pregnancy is often the major precipitating factor. The more sedentary lifestyles of many adults, and the resulting decrease in physical activity, may predispose them to obesity.

The age at which obesity develops provides important clues to the precise nature of the disorder. Early in life, the body grows rapidly and fat cells increase in both size and number. Later in life, as the rate of body growth slows, the production of fat cells tends to level

**TABLE 1-6.** *U.S. Government Recommended Weights for Men and Women*

| | WEIGHT IN POUNDS | |
| --- | --- | --- |
| Height | 19 to 34 years | 35 years and older |
| 5'0" | 97–128 | 108–138 |
| 5'1" | 101–132 | 111–143 |
| 5'2" | 104–137 | 115–148 |
| 5'3" | 107–141 | 119–152 |
| 5'4" | 111–146 | 122–157 |
| 5'5" | 114–150 | 126–162 |
| 5'6" | 118–155 | 130–167 |
| 5'7" | 121–160 | 134–172 |
| 5'8" | 125–164 | 138–178 |
| 5'9" | 129–169 | 142–183 |
| 5'10" | 132–174 | 146–188 |
| 5'11" | 136–179 | 151–194 |
| 6'0" | 140–184 | 155–199 |
| 6'1" | 144–189 | 159–205 |
| 6'2" | 148–195 | 164–210 |

Source: U.S. Department of Agriculture, U.S. Department of Health and Human Services.

off, but their size may enlarge to store excess energy. This leads to the conclusion that childhood-onset obesity is probably due to a greatly increased number of cells (called hypercellular or hyperplastic obesity), while adult-onset obesity is more likely the result of greatly enlarged fat cells (called hypertrophic obesity).

## FACTORS CONTRIBUTING TO OBESITY

It is also possible to classify obesity according to the factors responsible for its development. As will be discussed at greater length in chapter 2, the causes of obesity are varied and, in some cases, not fully understood.

Physical inactivity is one of the most important causes of obesity. Activity levels have significant impact on the body systems that control the storage, utilization, and deposition of energy (food).

Another important cause of obesity is diet. Overconsumption of high-fat, high-calorie foods is one of the chief dietary contributors to obesity.

Genetic factors are also believed to play a part in the development of obesity; however, the precise gene links are still unknown at the present time. There is growing evidence that genetics may have an influence on the body's tendency to store energy either as fat or as lean tissue. In addition, variations in metabolic processes, which could predispose one to obesity, may be inherited. Certain genetically linked disorders, such as Prader-Willi syndrome, involve appetite regulation abnormalities that can lead to obesity, but such conditions are very rare.

Other contributing factors include various endocrine dysfunctions, such as pituitary deficiency, adrenal disease, ovarian disease, or overproduction of insulin. Overall, however, endocrine abnormalities causing obesity are uncommon. Finally, a variety of social, economic, and psychological factors have been associated with the onset of obesity. Compared to upper income groups, people of lower socioeconomic status have elevated rates of obesity, even at very young ages. Poor nutrition may be responsible for much of this disparity, although such links are difficult to establish with any certainty.

# 2

# CAUSES OF
# OBESITY

The root causes of obesity, much like the very definition of obesity, are hotly debated by those who study
the disease. Acknowledging the complex, multifaceted
nature of the disorder, a 1992 editorial in the *New
England Journal of Medicine* even went so far as to say
". . . any statement nowadays that begins 'Obesity
is . . .' is apt to be wrong."[1]

It is possible to explain that obesity results from
excess energy intake and inadequate energy expenditure over an extended period of time. Beyond this simple explanatory statement, however, opinions diverge as
to the relative importance of factors that create the
imbalance between energy intake and expenditure. *JM for example*

A great deal of research has been aimed at the
genetic composition, metabolic function, nutritional
habits, and behavioral/lifestyle choices of obese patients. Psychological and environmental factors in the
development of obesity have also received considerable
attention.

All these elements likely play significant roles in the
development of obesity. However, not only is there
some controversy over the relative importance of the
various factors, but precise mechanisms may vary from

individual to individual, further complicating the task of determining a cause.

Given the uncertainties, most obesity experts agree that the condition is usually the result of complex interactions. Some of the most common causes of obesity will be discussed in this chapter.

## OVEREATING

It is easy to assume that if excess energy intake results in weight gain, then obesity must stem from chronic overeating. People of normal weight in particular, using their own experiences as a standard, may find such a hypothesis quite attractive. Media images further reinforce the idea that obese persons routinely consume mass quantities of food by depicting such individuals in the midst of smorgasbord-style feeding frenzies. As a result an impression persists that obesity is due primarily to gluttony.

But the connection between overeating and obesity is not necessarily so direct. First of all, the very term "overeating" is quite loose. Overeating may be defined as "the degree of food intake of a particular individual that brings in more food energy than is needed in order to maintain a given weight." But the same quantity of food intake may have very different effects from one individual to the next. As a result, persons of similar age, sex, and activity level may have hugely different food intake patterns without significant difference in body weight. Even after extended periods of restrictive dieting (1,000 or fewer calories per day), some people will not lose weight. Yet, they cannot rightly be accused of overeating.

Studies over the past twenty years generally support the position that obese persons consume no more calories than naturally lean individuals.[2,3] In some cases, obese persons have been observed to consume fewer calories than their normal-weight counterparts. A more likely dietary contributor to obesity is the overconsumption of high-fat foods. (This is discussed under Environmental Factors in this chapter.)

It must be noted that study techniques to assess food intake are not perfect. Many studies rely upon dietary diaries or the recollections of the participants. Other study results may be flawed by unusual eating patterns, such as bingeing. Nevertheless, most evidence[4] seems to suggest that overeating is not the primary cause of obesity.*

In rare cases, obesity may be caused by abnormalities in appetite regulation. The hypothalamus, a portion of the brain, controls the complex system of checks and balances that regulate appetite. If the hypothalamus is impaired, as in Prader-Willi syndrome, insatiable hunger may result.

## LIFESTYLE

Lifestyle choices have important implications for most aspects of human health, including weight regulation. Therefore, it is not surprising that one of the most significant contributors to the development of obesity is a sedentary, or inactive, lifestyle. Physical activity

---

* A highly publicized study reported in 1992 revealed that obese subjects may be inclined to underestimate their caloric intake and overestimate their energy expenditure.[4] The study authors pointed out that such discrepancies were not conscious attempts at deception, but rather the result of genuine misperceptions. The findings, readers were warned, "should not be misconstrued to mean that their obesity was simply a consequence of gluttony and sloth. Nonobese persons also underestimate their caloric intake."

stimulates increased metabolism, promoting the consumption of energy from food; its absence contributes to an energy imbalance that can eventually lead to excess weight gain.

A remarkably high number of people in the United States and most other affluent countries lead sedentary lifestyles. The explosive growth of technology has ushered in automation, eliminating much of the manual labor that once was a part of everyday living. A dazzling array of time-saving, easy-to-use consumer products, ranging from washing machines, vacuum cleaners, and food processors to remote control devices, leaf blowers, and automatic garage door openers, has made possible—even encouraged—sedentary lifestyles. But of all the gadgets and gimmicks that have influenced the shift toward physical inactivity, none has been more significant than the automobile. Routinely used for the shortest of errands or shopping trips, cars have made it possible for even the most sedentary people to get around.

The trend away from physical activity and toward idleness is not only an adult phenomenon. Many youngsters who might once have spent their spare time playing outside increasingly opt for indoor entertainment like watching television or playing computer games. (See Figure 2–1.)

Certainly, the advent of labor-saving equipment has its benefits. This can be seen very clearly, for example, in agricultural production, where, in the past forty years, technology has transformed an occupation once largely dependent on the physical strength of humans and animals to one that is almost completely mechanized. Such technical advances have helped boost the output of America's farms to the point where one Iowa farmer now produces enough food to feed more than

**FIGURE 2-1.** *Prevalence of Obesity in 12- to 17-year-old Adolescents Related to Hours of Daily Television Viewing.*

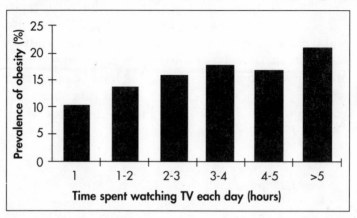

Some researchers have linked obesity in adolescents with time spent watching television. The relationship, though striking, is not well understood at the present time. It may be that TV watching is simply accompanied by increased consumption of snack foods and decreased rates of exercise. Or TV viewing may actually have some effect on emotional or metabolic function, resulting in excessive weight gain.

Source: M.D. Willard. "Obesity: Types and Treatments." *American Family Practitioner*, 43:2099, 1991.

two hundred fifty people.[5] In certain heavy industries, such as steel manufacturing, automated machinery now performs much of the most laborious and dangerous work once done by workers, thus reducing the likelihood of workplace injury or death.

As machinery has taken over much of the most backbreaking labor, people's caloric energy needs have been reduced. In many cases, however, diets needed to sustain one through the rigors of manual labor have not been changed to meet the lower energy requirements. Weight gain, and eventually obesity, is the usual result.

A regular regimen of moderate to rigorous exercise and dietary adjustments are effective ways to counter a sedentary lifestyle. Not only is exercise one of the most effective ways to prevent obesity, but it is also associated with an array of other positive health outcomes. According to the United States Public Health Service's *Healthy People 2000* report,

> *Regular physical activity can help to prevent and manage coronary heart disease, hypertension, noninsulin-dependent diabetes mellitus, osteoporosis, obesity, and mental health problems (e.g., depression, anxiety). Regular physical activity has also been associated with lower rates of colon cancer and stroke and may be linked to reduced back injury. On average, physically active people outlive those who are inactive. Regular physical activity can also help to maintain the functional independence of older adults and enhance the quality of life for people of all ages.*[6]

Unfortunately, few Americans seem to take such advice seriously. It is estimated that less than 10 percent of adults exercise at recommended levels.* While it might be expected that older people would cut down on physical activity, surveys show that inactivity has been increasing rapidly even among adolescents and young adults. Ironically, this inactivity occurs in spite of the

---

* In 1990, the United States Public Health Service issued recommendations calling for "exercise which involves large muscle groups in dynamic movement for periods of 20 minutes or longer, 3 or more days per week, and which is performed at an intensity of 60 percent or greater of an individual's cardiorespiratory capacity."

younger generation's ongoing love affair with athletic events. Some might say Americans are becoming a nation of sports enthusiasts whose workouts consist of little more than lifting, pointing, and pressing a television remote control unit.

## GENETIC FACTORS

At the present time, the influence of inherited factors on obesity is not entirely clear. Studies involving parents and their children, identical twins, brothers and sisters, and adoptive siblings have yielded varied results. Some identify a strong genetic effect while others conclude genetics played a relatively minor role in predicting obesity.

In supporting the genetic connection in obesity, investigators have reported that almost three-fourths of obese patients had an obese parent. However, it is exceedingly difficult to separate inherited factors from the more obvious behavioral and lifestyle conditions that are known to cause obesity. Still, the evidence is clear that having obese parents places one at increased risk of developing obesity, whatever the specific mechanisms may be.[7]

Genetic factors may have a considerable effect on a person's resting metabolic rate, the energy expended by the body at rest for purposes of respiration, circulation, digestion, and other basic life functions. A lower than normal resting metabolic rate predisposes one to obesity because the body consumes fewer calories for its maintenance.

Some research[8] seems to indicate that genetic coding may also affect body composition, thus making some individuals more susceptible to becoming obese. In a process called nutrient partitioning, the body stores excess energy either as fat or as lean (fat-free) tissue. If inherited qualities make a body prone to store nutrients as fat, rather than lean tissue, the result will be weight gain.

The task of identifying inherited causes of any disorder is formidable, but understanding the genetic aspects of obesity is made even more difficult by the fact that the term obesity is used to describe a number of very dissimilar conditions. For example, obesity characterized by fat accumulation in the abdominal region is quite different from obesity marked by excess fat in the buttocks and thighs. Assuming that inherited factors are at play, it is very likely that these different types of obesity have discrete genetic links. Therefore, proving the genetic connection will require identification of the precise genes that produce a specific form of obesity.

## ETHNICITY

Interesting genetic studies have been carried out to compare rates of obesity among certain ethnic groups. For example, the Pima Indians, a native American population known to have extremely high rates of obesity, have been the subject of a great many investigations.[9,10] About two-thirds of the women and one-half of the men in this tribe are obese. Since the Pima have participated in long-term weight studies, researchers have been able to determine that obesity in this group is familial. However, the relative importance of genetics and environmental factors has not been positively determined.

Obesity is also very prevalent in other minority populations, particularly African American and Hispanic populations. Females in these ethnic groups are at higher risk of obesity, especially in late adolescence and adulthood. There may be genetic factors predisposing these groups to obesity; however, other factors such as physical inactivity, higher food energy intake, and earlier age at first childbirth may also be important.[11]

---

## ENVIRONMENTAL FACTORS

When considering environmental factors contributing to obesity, the totality of conditions that form the individual's milieu must be considered. These may include the entire range of behavioral, dietary, social, and economic conditions that surround an individual throughout his or her life. The amount and type of food routinely available in a household, the methods in which foods are prepared for meals, family attitudes and behaviors regarding snacking and physical activity, and attitudes regarding the acceptability of greater body weight are some environmental factors, as they contribute to the environment in which an individual lives. Depending on which elements are present, which are stressed, and which are ignored, the interplay of these environmental factors could point one toward obesity.

Behaviors and attitudes learned early in life may be some of the strongest indicators of adult body type. These attitudes and beliefs become the lifelong standards by which a person regulates his or her own behavior.

Whereas genetic factors leading to obesity are very difficult to pinpoint, environmental factors are usually much more apparent. A person's eating and exercise habits can be easily monitored, for instance, to determine what foods are eaten, how foods are prepared, what time of day meals are consumed, the frequency and intensity of physical activity, and so on. This kind of information is very useful in the treatment or prevention of obesity.

Among the environmental constituents of obesity, the high-fat diet eaten by many Americans is believed to be a particularly powerful predictor of the disorder. While obesity has been increasing in the United States throughout this century, the caloric intake of the average American has declined. However, the percentage of calories derived from fat has jumped markedly—from about 32 percent in 1910 to about 40 percent in 1990.[12]

When combined with the increasingly sedentary lifestyle, high-fat low-fiber diets quickly place one in positive energy balance (an overabundance of calories, which are then stored as fat). To reduce fat intake, the National Academy of Sciences and other health organizations recommend eating more foods rich in complex carbohydrates (vegetables and grains) and less fatty foods (luncheon meat, the skin on chicken, and food that is fried). Eating fruit instead of fatty pastry for dessert would also help to decrease fat intake.*

Environmental factors also include socioeconomic conditions. Some research indicates that dietary habits (along with many other health habits) correlate closely with socioeconomic status: groups with higher rates of college education or higher income typically eat healthier foods and are more likely to practice recommended weight management techniques. Specifically, they tend to consume more fruits and vegetables, more high-fiber foods, and less high-fat meats.[13] As a result, rates of obesity are generally lower among these groups and higher among economically disadvantaged groups.[14]

Another cause of obesity that might be described as

---

* Five or more servings (½ cup each) of fruits and vegetables each day is suggested. Six or more servings of foods rich in complex carbohydrates like breads, pasta, and cereals is suggested.

environmental is the use of certain drugs—prescription or otherwise—that are known to affect body weight and the accumulation of fat. For instance, considerable weight gain is one side effect of some drugs used to treat chronic immunologic diseases and depression.* Doctors treating obese patients for these health conditions must be very cautious about prescribing medications that could exacerbate existing weight problems.

Some researchers even suggest that environmental factors such as the seasons, geographic location, population density, and increased television viewing may cause obesity.[15,16] It is conceivable that any of these elements could influence an individual's bodily processes (particularly metabolism), thus potentially predisposing him or her to obesity.

## PSYCHOLOGICAL FACTORS

For many years, psychoanalysts and nutritionists assumed that obesity was either a result of, or an indication of, underlying psychiatric problems, such as depression or anxiety. More recently, however, a number of studies have shown that obese persons do not necessarily experience greater psychiatric disturbance than do normal-weight persons.[17]

There is some evidence that obese individuals who seek treatment for their disease have higher rates of psychiatric problems than the general population; how-

---

* That drugs effect body weight can also be seen in the use of nicotine, the active ingredient in tobacco. Just one cigarette can raise the metabolic rate by as much as 15 percent, which in turn accelerates energy consumption and weight loss. As a result, smokers typically weigh less than nonsmokers, and many people who stop smoking are prone to weight gain.

ever, even these levels are about the same as for other patients undergoing surgical or medical treatment.[18] (It is not unusual for persons under a doctor's care to experience anxiety about their vulnerability and their physical health.)

As one research group concluded, "There appear to be very few personality characteristics unique to obese persons."[19] On balance, obesity is not thought to be caused by psychiatric disorders, nor is there evidence that the mental health of obese people differs substantially from that of the general population.[20]

However, research consistently suggests that certain patterns of behavior and psychological factors are more prevalent among obese individuals than normal-weight persons. For example, binge eating (also known as bulimia), in which a person eats great quantities of food in a very short period of time, is relatively common among obese people. Estimates of binge eating among obese individuals undergoing treatment range from 23 percent to 82 percent.[21] (Although binge eating is commonly thought of as a behavioral problem, the American Psychiatric Association places it on its list of mental disorders.) In compulsive eating disorders like bulimia, a psychological need, rather than hunger, is the motivation for eating.

Most health professionals today see obesity resulting from the interaction of multiple factors, including certain predisposing genetic traits, an environment replete with great quantities of food (much of it high in fat content), and reduced demands for physical activity.

"The rising incidence of obesity in the Western world during the past century is due, to some extent, to those improvements in nutrition and hygiene that are also reflected in trends in menarche [onset of menstruation] at an earlier age and greater adult stature," according to one physician observer.[22] Simply put, many of the same advances that have helped to enhance the quality of modern life—a stable and abundant food supply, labor-saving machinery, and so on—also put people at risk of a serious health problem such as obesity. Given this situation, in order to avoid excessive weight gain, one must make concerted efforts to increase physical activity and decrease caloric intake.

While it is generally not possible to alter inherited characteristics, obesity is also determined by lifestyle and environmental factors. And by modifying these elements, it may be possible for people to avoid the conditions that lead to obesity.

# 3
# HEALTH CONSEQUENCES OF OBESITY

In addition to many practical and social difficulties, obesity also increases a person's risks of serious illness. Many of the illnesses associated with obesity, such as heart disease, diabetes, and some forms of cancer, are extremely grave and often fatal. In most cases, people who are severely obese over a long period of time are most likely to suffer from such diseases.

Many other troublesome, but usually nonfatal, conditions also accompany obesity. Among the most common are hypertension (high blood pressure), gallbladder disease, reproductive problems, and sleep disorders. Osteoarthritis, resulting in severe joint pain in areas such as the knees, lower back, ankles, feet, and hips, also is common, as is the development of varicose veins.

Beyond these physical impairments, obesity is also associated with a variety of psychological conditions. These disorders, although not usually life-threatening, do represent real personal challenges. Some psychological obstacles are minimal; others are serious enough to interfere with the performance of basic daily routines.

This chapter will examine some of the most common health consequences associated with obesity.

## CARDIOVASCULAR DISEASE

A primary health consequence of obesity is cardiovascular disease (CVD), a disease that affects the heart and the body's circulatory system, consisting of arteries and veins.

Severely obese persons are believed to be at significantly higher risk of developing CVDs, including stroke, hypertension, congestive heart failure, and coronary heart disease. Some studies indicate that obese people are twice as likely as normal-weight people to suffer from hypertension and stroke.

Hypertension is one of the most common health problems in America, and obesity dramatically increases one's chances of developing this condition. Many doctors believe that hypertension develops in obese persons because the heart and circulatory system are under increased strain to move blood throughout a greatly enlarged body, but this explanation is not proved. Hypertension is often not diagnosed for many years, during which time it can inflict considerable damage, particularly to the structure of the blood vessels. If left untreated, high blood pressure can lead to stroke, heart failure, and severe kidney and eye damage. Mild hypertension may be controlled by weight loss; otherwise, a range of medications is available.

Another serious form of CVD is atherosclerosis, a disease in which fat deposits accumulate on the walls of blood vessels. Over time, these deposits build, thus narrowing the channel through which blood flows. This narrowing of the arteries restricts the delivery of blood to tissues throughout the body, including the heart, brain, kidneys, and the various muscle groups. In severe atherosclerosis, an artery may become completely obstructed, resulting in a stroke or heart attack. Although atherosclerosis affects most adults to some degree, obesity is believed to aggravate the condition considerably. High blood pressure and diabetes, other conditions that commonly accompany obesity, also exacerbate arterial narrowing.

Several studies also show that heart function is adversely affected by obesity.[1,2] Coronary disease and congestive heart failure are two of the most common—and most deadly—CVD conditions that have been attributed to excess body weight.

Cardiovascular diseases are the leading cause of death in the United States and among the nation's most expensive health problems. According to the American Heart Association, the cost of cardiovascular conditions in the United States will amount to 128 billion dollars in 1994.[3] The high cost of medications, surgical procedures, hospital services, and lost productivity due to disability all add to the enormity of the bill. Certainly, factors other than obesity (notably, cigarette smoking) contribute to CVD. But obesity is a significant risk factor, and one that can be prevented and controlled.

The precise connection between obesity and CVD is still uncertain. For one thing, although the U.S. population (especially men), has been getting heavier over the past twenty years, death rates from CVD have been decreasing. This paradox interests many public health researchers. While acknowledging "confusion over the complex relationship between obesity and CVD," the authors of one important study concluded that "leanness and avoidance of weight gain before middle age are advisable goals in the prevention of CVD for most American men and women."[4] The authors also suggested that medical treatments should be accompanied by weight loss efforts.

# DIABETES MELLITUS

Noninsulin-dependent diabetes mellitus (NIDDM) is a condition that is characterized by an insufficiency of insulin, the hormone that enables the body to store and utilize sugars. Untreated, this condition leads to abnormal weight loss and fatigue. Obesity is the most significant risk factor for the development of this disease; adult onset of NIDDM is five times more common among obese people.

Usually in NIDDM, insulin is produced, but not in great enough amounts to meet the body's needs. The excess weight present in obese persons only worsens the shortfall. Some people who suffer from NIDDM actually produce "normal" amounts of insulin, but still have an insufficiency because their bodies are resistant to the effects of insulin. Weight loss, oral medications, and special dietary practices are usually sufficient to control NIDDM.

Diabetes is a very widespread problem—about 10 million Americans are diagnosed diabetics and another 5 million are believed to have milder forms of the disease without knowing it. About nine out of ten diabetics suffer from NIDDM as opposed to another, more serious, form called insulin-dependent diabetes, which must be treated with insulin injections.

Diabetes also predisposes one to other health problems. Male diabetics have about twice the normal risk of coronary artery disease and female diabetics about five times the normal risk.[5] Ulcers on the feet are also possible because diabetes frequently leads to blood vessel damage. Other complications related to diabetes include kidney, eye, and nerve damage. These problems usually reduce the life expectancy of people with NIDDM.

# CANCER

The first studies linking obesity and cancer were done in the 1940s.[6] Over the years, there have been a number of shifts in opinion regarding the relationship. At the present time, it is thought that excessive weight is associated with increased rates of cancer, particularly in certain sites such as the colon, rectum, and prostate in men, and the cervix, ovary, breast, endometrium, and gallbladder in women.

A large, long-term study by the American Cancer Society also found increased rates of kidney, stomach, and uterine cancers among obese persons. Overall, obese men had a 33 percent greater risk and obese women had a 55 percent greater risk of cancer than their normal-weight counterparts. These findings prompted the American Cancer Society to observe, "For people who are obese, weight reduction is a good way to lower cancer risk."[7]

A discussion of obesity's relationship to cancer must touch on the role of diet. The American Cancer Society's "Guidelines on Diet, Nutrition, and Cancer" recommends seven dietary practices designed to lower the risk of developing cancer:

- Maintain a desirable body weight.

- Eat a varied diet.

- Include a variety of both vegetables and fruits in the daily diet.

- Eat more high-fiber foods, such as whole-grain cereals, legumes, vegetables, and fruits.

- Cut down on total fat intake.

- Limit consumption of alcoholic beverages, if you drink at all.

- Limit consumption of salt-cured, smoked, and nitrite-preserved foods.

In highlighting the importance of sound nutrition, the report also states: "It is estimated that about one-third of the annual 500,000 deaths from cancer in the United States, including the most common sites such as breast, colon, and prostate, may be attributed to undesirable dietary practices."[8]

Other organizations and government agencies frequently issue dietary recommendations, with or without reference to the relationship between eating habits and cancer. Sometimes the information contained in these reports can appear contradictory or, at the very least, confusing. However, most responsible dietary guidelines for cancer prevention have two basic principles: (1) eat a wide variety of foods, and (2) avoid obesity.

Despite enormous effort and investment, determining the cause of cancer has proven very difficult for researchers. Each form of cancer is a unique disease entity, not just a slight variant of one common ailment. Different cancers exhibit different cellular characteristics, progress at different speeds, metastasize (spread) to different locations, and respond to different therapies. The risk profile, which is the set of circumstances that place an individual at risk of developing cancer, can be extremely complex. Unique environmental exposures might explain the development of a malignancy, genetic factors might be at play, a combination of known and unknown elements could be the cause. Given all the conceivable causative agents, isolating a specific one with absolute certainty can be practically impossible.

**TABLE 3-1.** *Health Problems Related to Obesity*

| | |
|---|---|
| Cardiovascular Disease | Accelerated atherosclerosis<br>Angina<br>Congestive heart failure<br>Coronary heart disease<br>Hypertension<br>Stroke |
| Cancer | Prostate<br>Colon<br>Breast<br>Ovary<br>Cervix<br>Endometrium<br>Kidney<br>Stomach |
| Diabetes mellitus | |
| Hyperlipidemia<br>(elevated concentrations of fat in blood) | |
| Gallbladder disease | |
| Lung disease | |
| Osteoarthritis | |
| Psychological distress | |
| Reproductive disorders | Infertility<br>Menstrual dysfunction |
| Sleep apnea | |
| Varicose veins | |

Yet, in light of the fact that there is such great public interest in cancer, organizations and agencies concerned with this disease are expected to issue recommendations. Responsible advice about cancer risk reduction is based on the best available scientific evidence, but such advice may be confirmed or disproved by subsequent research.

## MUSCULOSKELETAL PROBLEMS

Because of their extreme body weight, obese persons frequently develop musculoskeletal problems, including arthritis and other painful joint disorders. The excess weight puts added stress on major weight-bearing joints, such as the hips, knees, spine, and ankles. One of the most common joint disorders to afflict the obese is osteoarthritis.

In healthy joints, the ends of the bones that come together are sheathed in cartilage, which serves as a cushion. The joint is also lubricated by fluid and protected by surrounding bands of tissue called ligaments. When osteoarthritis develops, the cartilage deteriorates and the joint's natural cushion is lost. Abnormal bone growth may also occur, resulting in the appearance of bony lumps around the affected joint.

Osteoarthritis is caused by excessive wear and tear to the given joint and is marked by pain, swelling, and a loss of flexibility. Many older people naturally develop osteoarthritis, but obese persons typically experience its debilitating effects at much younger ages. Weight loss will not reverse osteoarthritis, but it will help to relieve joint pain and is therefore a valuable addition to other therapies. Treatments for this disease include the use of heating pads, range-of-motion exercises, and muscle strengthening activities.

## REPRODUCTIVE DISORDERS

Evidence suggests a definite link between body fat and reproductive health, with both excess and insufficient fat negatively affecting reproduction. In the female body, sufficient fat appears to be necessary for normal functioning of the reproductive cycle. Thus, under-weight adolescent females often do not experience menarche, while many adult women with inadequate body weight fail to have regular menstrual cycles.

Reproductive disorders also result in the obese. The sexual functioning of females appears to be adversely affected by excess fat. While about 2.5 percent of normal-weight women fail to ovulate normally, that number increases to more than 8 percent for severely obese females. A gynecological study found that as many as 58 percent of women complaining of men-strual dysfunction could be classified as obese. On the other hand, this study found that only 13 percent of women with normal menstrual cycles fit the re-searchers' definition of obesity.[9] While other factors may have influenced these individuals' fertility prob-lems, obesity is generally recognized as an important contributing factor.

Women suffering both obesity and reproductive disorders show specific endocrine (hormonal) abnor-malities. Many such women exhibit increased levels of androgens, which are male sex hormones. The elevated presence of androgens interferes with normal female sexual function. In a great many cases, no other treat-ment than weight loss is required to reduce androgen levels and restore fertility.

Obese men also face reproductive dilemmas. Obe-sity is associated with male impotence and reduced sperm production. In both men and women, extreme obesity can also be a serious physical impediment to sexual intercourse. In such cases, simple weight loss is the most effective treatment to restore normal sexual function.

## PSYCHOLOGICAL ASPECTS

For many years, there was an assumption that obesity was either caused by or indicated underlying psychiatric problems, such as depression or an inability to cope with stress. More recent study suggests that factors once believed to cause obesity are more likely consequences of the condition.

In addition, psychological differences between obese individuals and those of normal weight include perceptions about body image and attitudes toward weight and eating. Body image has been defined as the "perception of one's body size and appearance and the emotional response to these perceptions."[10] Typically, obese individuals are less accurate than normal-weight persons in estimating their size and appearance.* On average, obese people overestimate their own body size by 6 to 12 percent and are three times more likely to do so than non-obese subjects.

Some observers believe this tendency of obese persons to exaggerate their bodily proportions is part of a pattern. Strong negative reactions to their own physical appearance often develop into an "overwhelming preoccupation with one's obesity, often to the exclusion of any other personal characteristics," according to one prominent psychiatric study.[11] Depending on the fre-

---

* In body image evaluations patients are usually asked to identify drawings or pictures that correlate with their perception of their own body. Using modern video technology this can also be done through the manipulation of the patient's own picture displayed on a television screen.

quency and the intensity of these perceptions, they may crowd out more positive feelings that are important to a healthy self-image.

Many obese persons also appear to be particularly anxious on issues directly related to weight and eating. They may, for instance, be much more self-conscious about the amount of food they eat during a meal, and feel more depressed about their appearance than normal-weight persons. This contrasts with surveys of their depression, assertiveness, and self-consciousness on topics unrelated to weight and eating, which indicate virtually no differences between obese and non-obese groups.

Finally, there are longer-term psychological aspects of obesity, especially among persons attempting to bring their weight under control. Obesity is, in most cases, a lifelong problem involving genetic and biological factors and significant long-term weight reduction is the exception rather than the rule. Unrealistic expectations of fast and easy weight loss, widely promoted by "quick fix" diets and "miracle" gadgets in magazine and television advertisements, encourage false hope among those who desire to lose weight and discourage unsuccessful patients. In addition, weight regain, a very frequent occurrence among obese patients who have had some initial success in losing weight, can have serious negative psychological effects. Feelings of failure, guilt, and hopelessness are common among those who regain weight after having struggled to lose it.

One person who struggled with obesity described the initial thrill of weight loss brought on by improved mobility, flattering remarks from friends, and the ability to fit into clothes long kept in storage.

"I suppose there was quite a lot of ego involved," he said. "Not the least of the pleasures I enjoyed were the compliments of friends and colleagues who told me how good I looked after having lost so much weight."

Inevitably, the novelty of his leanness faded and the reinforcing compliments from others ceased. The continuing need to monitor calorie intake and to forego the pleasures of certain favorite foods also became tiresome. Over time, he regained a considerable amount of the weight he had worked hard to lose.

Physicians treating obese individuals for psychological distress (whether or not such distress is associated with obesity) also face significant challenges. Some of the most commonly used antidepressant medications actually increase appetite and promote weight gain. Furthermore, since statistics indicate that most obese individuals do not achieve and maintain long-term weight loss, doctors must help their obese patients set realistic goals and think of obesity as a chronic illness for which a "cure" is not always possible. Rather, successful management of the disease means limiting the health consequences of obesity and preventing the emergence of other health problems secondary to obesity, such as osteoarthritis.

Doctors can also help obese patients counter some of the discouragement likely to be felt when weight reduction targets are not met by encouraging the development of other goals in addition to weight loss, such as decreasing blood pressure or improving exercise habits. In this way, it is possible for the patient to both experience the positive feelings associated with meeting a target and decrease the preoccupation with weight and dieting.

## WEIGHT CYCLING

Some recent evidence suggests that the negative health effects of obesity are not necessarily limited to conditions of excess weight. Patterns of weight loss and gain might also precipitate diseases.

Many obese people make multiple attempts at weight reduction that are unsuccessful. So-called "weight cycling," the fluctuation in body weight that results from a pattern of weight loss and subsequent regain, has been associated with serious health problems that can affect a person, including coronary heart disease.

A recent examination of weight cycling among participants in the Framingham Heart Study* showed that fluctuations in body weight correlated with higher rates of coronary heart disease and higher death rates.[12] The investigators conducting the study acknowledged the difficulty of drawing firm conclusions about the links between weight fluctuation and longevity, but suggested their results have significance for the millions of Americans trying to lose weight by dieting.

"If dieting emerges as a major factor in body-weight fluctuation, it may be important to evaluate further the public health implications of current weight-loss practices," caution the authors. "Approximately 50 percent of American women and 25 percent of American men are dieting at any time, and many diets are unsuccessful." Therefore, it is all the more important to teach obese persons how to maintain their hard-earned weight losses. Physicians and others involved in the treatment of obesity must also focus on strategies that prevent relapses.

---

* Since 1948, more than 5,000 male and female residents of Framingham, Massachusetts, have participated in a long-term study of heart disease. The study involves physical examinations every two years. Many investigators have used data collected from his group to study other aspects of human health, including obesity.

## OTHER DISORDERS

Among the many other health problems related to obesity, one of the most frequent is a condition called sleep apnea, in which breathing temporarily stops during sleep. The disruption caused by recurrent episodes of sleep apnea prevents an individual from entering deep levels of sleep, which are necessary for normal daytime functioning.

Normally, during sleep the muscles in the throat stay tense, which keeps the airway open and permits inhalation. In sleep apnea, these muscles relax and the walls of the throat collapse, cutting off the flow of air into the lungs. After 20 to 30 seconds, the sleeper rouses, the throat opens, air exchange resumes, and the cycle begins again. The excess weight of an obese person, particularly if it is distributed largely to the upper body, may be responsible for collapsing the airway. Weight reduction will correct this disorder in 90 percent of patients.

Other obesity-related health problems include hernias, skin irritation from constant rubbing (as with inner thighs), inability to keep oneself clean, fatigue, labored breathing, and immobility.

# 4

# TREATMENT OPTIONS FOR OBESITY

Despite impressive research gains and the introduction of some promising new therapies, rates of long-term weight loss for obese individuals remain disappointingly low. Only about 10 percent of obese individuals achieve permanent reversal of their condition.[1]

The extreme difficulty in managing obesity can be traced to the fact that there are still many missing pieces of the puzzle. As Dr. Jules Hirsch of Rockefeller University noted, "The greatest barrier to the treatment of obesity remains our incomplete understanding of the complex genetic, developmental, and psychosocial influences that lead to obesity."[2]

Treatment options for the management of obesity range from a prescription of very low-calorie diets and physical exercise to certain surgical procedures. Diet and exercise are considered conservative treatments, while options such as surgery are considered aggressive treatments.

According to recent research, drug therapy may be an important tool in treating obesity. To date, however, drug treatment (mainly appetite suppressant medications) remains a rather controversial option.

Fat cells have an extremely long life span. Changes in body fat may shrink the size of individual fat cells, but the total number of fat cells remains largely unchanged. "Even marked and prolonged weight loss does not decrease the number of fat cells," writes Dr. George Bray.[3]

This information has important implications for the treatment of obese persons. Since the total number of fat cells may be relatively constant, it is exceedingly difficult to achieve and maintain weight reduction, especially for those suffering from hyperplastic obesity, the form of obesity caused by a greatly increased number of fat cells.

Given the existence of a stable number of excess fat cells, the only practicable weight loss technique would be to shrink the size of those cells below normal. However, body processes appear to resist such a solution, tending to return cells to normal size. Since it is so difficult to lose fat cells, it is easy to understand how long-term weight reduction becomes such a daunting prospect for many obese persons.

## CONSERVATIVE TREATMENT OPTIONS

In most cases, conservative approaches are the first to be applied in the treatment of obesity. Conservative treatment plans usually emphasize modification of eating habits and increased physical activity to achieve desired weight reductions. In addition, concerted efforts to bring about long-term lifestyle changes, improve negative attitudes, enhance stress management skills, develop coping techniques, and de-emphasize the role of food in the obese subject's life are also important components of a conservative treatment plan.

## BEHAVIORAL MODIFICATION

Taken as a whole, the wide-reaching plan to promote the adoption of new daily habits and a healthier lifestyle is called behavioral modification. Probably the most widely used technique to achieve weight loss, some form of behavioral modification is integrated into most obesity treatment plans, including such well-known commercial diet programs as Weight Watchers, Diet Center, and NutriSystem. Even if aggressive treatment options such as surgery are employed, behavioral modification remains an important part of the long-term treatment plan.

The difficulty of establishing meaningful behavioral modification and continuing it over the long term is perhaps the primary reason for the failure of most obese people to achieve and maintain significant weight losses.

Behavior therapy usually takes place in group sessions, with about ten to fifteen patients meeting with a specially trained therapist. Depending on the program, the group may meet for about one or two hours per week for a period of ten to twenty weeks. Most successful behavioral therapy programs include long-term (at least one year) follow-up. This allows patients to continue to monitor their weight after the formal treatment sessions cease. Table 4–1 on pages 64 and 65 lists some specific techniques commonly used in behavioral modification programs.

In most cases, the components of behavioral modifications programs include:

*Self-monitoring.* Patients keep a daily log to assess eating and exercise behavior. The log includes information on what, when, and where they eat, and may also include notes on the social situations surrounding the eating event.

*Stimulus Control.* Steps are taken to eliminate or reduce patients' exposure to food or the cues that are commonly associated with eating. For instance, food is stored out of sight, eating times and locations are strictly limited, and activities associated with unapproved eating habits (such as watching television) are curtailed. In addition, all eating routines are examined to identify behaviors that could lead to excess consumption.

*Reinforcement.* Simple techniques are devised to reward attainment of a weight-loss goal. For example, a patient may purchase a new piece of clothing or a new music album as a reward for complying with the specified eating plan. This positive reinforcement provides stimulus to continue with a difficult weight-loss program.

*Nutrition.* In addition to limiting caloric intake, most successful behavioral modification programs teach patients some basic information about nutrition, i.e., limiting salt and fat intake, the importance of eating a balanced diet, and so on. Knowledge about good nutrition not only helps to bring about desired weight reductions, but also is an important element in overall good health.

*Exercise.* Exercise has multiple beneficial effects, including calorie consumption and positive psychological consequences. Exercise is also a useful diversion from routines that involve eating. Exercise can be incorporated into a daily routine (walking up a flight of stairs instead of taking the elevator, for instance) or implemented as a specific fitness program. For all obese patients, any exercise program must be approved by a doctor.

*Social Support.* An obese patient's support network, consisting of friends, family, and co-workers, can be a potent force for change. By encouraging the obese person to continue with the behavioral modification program and by avoiding the suggestion of behaviors that will undermine those efforts, a personal support system can contribute to successful weight management.

*Cognitive Change.* To overcome the many negative stereotypes about obese individuals, and to improve self-image, obese patients must develop new attitudes. By coming to see themselves as worthwhile persons struggling to cope with a very difficult health problem, obese patients are more likely to be motivated to succeed and to accept occasional failures.

Depending on the degree of obesity, the goal of conservative treatment may or may not involve achieving healthy body weight. For instance, in cases of extreme obesity (BMI of 45 or greater), the main objective may be simply to reduce the amount of excess body weight and body fat to more manageable levels. Even modest weight reductions can be expected to positively affect an obese person's functioning and minimize many health risks. It is also likely that moderate weight losses in severely obese patients will be more easily maintained than drastic reductions.

Conservative treatment programs differ, depending on the age, size, and activity level of each individual. A basic regimen may limit the patient to about 1,000 to 1,500 calories per day. The program may also require exercise that consumes an additional five calories per pound per day. Following such a program, an obese individual could expect to lose an average of one or two pounds a week.

Achieving weight loss through conservative techniques and maintaining such reductions over the long term requires great effort and, often, the assistance of a

**TABLE 4–1.** *Techniques in a Comprehensive Behavioral Modification Program*

## LIFESTYLE TECHNIQUES

1. Keep an eating diary
2. Maximize awareness of eating
3. Examine patterns in eating
4. Prevent automatic eating
5. Identify triggers for eating
6. Weigh yourself regularly
7. Keep a weight graph
8. Do nothing else while eating
9. Follow an eating schedule
10. Eat in one place
11. Do not clean your plate
12. Put your fork down between bites
13. Shop on a full stomach
14. Shop from a list
15. Buy foods that require preparation
16. Keep problem (high-sugar, high salt) foods out of sight
17. Keep healthy foods visible
18. Serve and eat one portion at a time
19. Use alternatives to eating
20. Plan in advance for high-risk situations (e.g., social situations where food will be available)

## EXERCISE TECHNIQUES

1. Keep an exercise diary
2. Understand the benefits of exercise
3. Increase walking opportunities
4. Increase lifestyle activity
5. Use stairs whenever possible
6. Know the calorie values of exercise
7. Choose and use programmed activity
8. Always warm up and cool down
9. Experiment with jogging, cycling, aerobics

## ATTITUDE TECHNIQUES

1. Weigh advantages and disadvantages of dieting
2. Realize complex causes of obesity
3. Distinguish hunger from cravings
4. Set realistic goals
5. Focus on behavior rather than weight
6. Banish imperatives from vocabulary
7. Be aware of high-risk situations
8. Outlast urges to eat
9. Cope positively with slips and lapses

## RELATIONSHIP TECHNIQUES

1. Identify and select a partner who will help you
2. Tell your partner how to help
3. Make specific and positive requests of partner
4. Reward your partner
5. Do not shop alone without partner (or)
6. Have partner do shopping for you
7. Exercise with partner
8. Use pleasurable partner activities

## NUTRITION TECHNIQUES

1. Eat less than 1200 calories per day (not recommended for everyone)
2. Be aware of calorie values of food
3. Know the basic food groups: bread, cereal, grains and pasta; vegetables; fruits; milk, yogurt, and cheese; meat, poultry, fish, dry beans, eggs, and nuts; fats, oils, sweets
4. Eat a balanced diet
5. Include adequate protein and carbohydrates in diet
6. Limit fat to 30 percent of total calories, with saturated fats making up less than 10 percent of the intake
7. Make low-calorie foods appetizing
8. Consume adequate vitamins
9. Increase fiber in diet

Adapted from Brownell, KD: Behavior management of obesity. *The Medical Clinics of North America* 73:185, 1989.

medical team. Physicians, nurses, dietitians, and social workers all may be important at different stages of the therapy. Each of these professionals can help an obese patient confront the physical, behavioral, and psychological barriers to weight loss. Since each obese person faces unique challenges, ranging from individual differences in metabolic rate to certain psychological hurdles, the treatment plan must be customized to meet each patient's specific needs.

## VERY-LOW-CALORIE DIETS

One treatment approach that has gained enormous popularity in recent years is the very-low-calorie diet (VLCD). This is a regimen that involves drastic reductions in caloric intake to produce rapid and substantial weight loss. For the moderately to severely obese person receiving proper guidance from a physician, the VLCD can be one of the most effective conservative treatment options.

The VLCD as a treatment for obesity was attempted as early as 1929, but doubts about its safety lingered. The reputation of the VLCD was badly damaged in the 1970s when so-called "liquid protein diets" attracted great attention. Thousands of people —many without adequate medical advice—enthusiastically tried these liquid diets, unaware that their poor composition resulted in severe malnutrition. The consequences were extremely grave. The Food and Drug Administration and the Centers for Disease Control estimate that these low-quality liquid protein diets caused the deaths of about sixty people.[4]

In contrast to these earlier low-calorie weight-loss programs, current VLCDs that provide-high quality protein and are administered under appropriate medical supervision are believed to be safe and effective.

The typical VLCD consists of about 400 to 800

calories per day, in contrast to a normal diet of about 2,500 to 3,500 calories per day. This extreme reduction in calories creates a large energy deficit which in turn results in dramatic weight loss. Over the course of the usual twelve- to fifteen-week VLCD program, patients can lose forty to fifty pounds. Longer programs of up to twenty-five weeks can produce weight losses in the range of sixty to seventy pounds, but many physicians discourage VLCDs of such extended duration. Extremely obese patients may be advised by their doctor to go through more than one cycle of VLCD-induced weight loss.

The drastic weight reductions achieved while a patient is on a VLCD may also be accompanied by undesirable side effects; therefore, such patients must be monitored closely. One frequent side effect of VLCDs is the formation of gallstones. The longer the weight-reduction program continues, the greater the risk.

It is especially important that weight lost during the period of the VLCD (or any by other method, for that matter) be primarily adipose tissue, rather than lean body mass.* An individual's nitrogen balance is an indirect gauge of the ratio of lean body mass loss to adipose tissue loss. Balanced nitrogen levels are usually equated with preservation of lean body mass, while negative balances indicate loss of lean body mass. High protein content in restricted-calorie diets is used to preserve lean body mass and maintain nitrogen balance.

While VLCDs are generally believed to be successful in achieving substantial weight loss, there are some problems associated with this technique. One problem

---

* Studies indicate that obese individuals protect lean body mass much more effectively than normal-weight individuals during restricted calorie dieting. Because they are losing mostly fat, the composition of their weight loss is considered much healthier.

relates to the VLCD's use of liquid formulas rather than solid foods. Although modern formulations can provide adequate nutrition, they cannot simulate real food in many ways that are important to long-term weight control. Specifically, formulations do nothing to help obese patients develop proper habits and attitudes relating to food: learning how to select appropriate foods at the grocery store, using healthy preparation methods, limiting portion sizes, and eating at a relaxed pace. So, although behavior modification is an important part of permanent weight management, liquid formula diets do not typically promote this component.

As Dr. F. Xavier Pi-Sunyer of the Obesity Research Center at St. Luke's/Roosevelt Hospital Center in New York City stated in a 1992 review of very-low-calorie diet programs: "Despite the statements made that behavior modification is part of VLCD programs, the truth of the matter is that this is not possible. One cannot modify behavior towards food without eating food. The VLCD is a way around the behavior."[5]

At a cost of about $2,000, VLCDs have also been criticized on economic grounds. Not only is the formula quite expensive, which effectively limits it to higher income groups, but because the sale of formula is the most lucrative part of many weight loss centers' business, these programs may neglect other important aspects crucial to permanent weight reduction, such as exercise and instruction in behavioral techniques.

Finally, because of the very serious risks associated with VLCDs, all such programs must be closely guided by a qualified medical professional. The decision to recommend a VLCD for an obese individual depends upon many factors, including the patient's age, sex, degree of obesity, and the presence of coexisting health problems. Once a patient begins the VLCD, the doctor must remain involved, setting appropriate weight reduction targets, determining the duration of the VLCD, and monitoring nitrogen balance. In addition, dosages of medications such as insulin need to be adjusted as weight loss progresses. No one should undertake a VLCD without the approval and careful supervision of a doctor.

Unfortunately, most research indicates that conservative treatment approaches do not enjoy great success. Perhaps the primary reason for failure is the inability of obese patients to endure the sustained program of food restriction and increased exercise required to produce significant weight loss. The Surgeon General's Report on Nutrition and Health, for example, advises a nine- to sixteen-month program of good nutrition, exercise, and lifestyle adjustments for obese persons. Dietary restrictions for an individual who is 100 pounds over ideal body weight could easily stretch on for more than three months. Such lengthy programs require tremendous commitment, motivation, and discipline—qualities all too often lacking in normal-weight individuals as well as obese patients.

When conservative treatments fail, many obese persons are recommended for more aggressive treatments, including surgical intervention. These options are discussed in the following section.

## AGGRESSIVE TREATMENT OPTIONS

If a severely obese individual fails to achieve and maintain significant weight loss through conservative measures, he or she may be advised to consider a surgical procedure.

Surgical intervention is used almost exclusively to treat cases of severe obesity, that is, patients with BMI greater than 35 or 40. In 1991, the National Institutes of Health issued a report stating: "Patients whose body mass index exceeds 40 may be considered for surgery if they strongly desire substantial weight loss because obesity severely impairs the quality of their lives."[6] Less severe obesity is usually treated with nonsurgical methods, although the NIH report suggested that individuals with BMI of 35 to 40 consider surgery if they also suffer from other high-risk conditions like cardiopulmonary disease, uncontrolled diabetes, hypertension, or sleep apnea. Because of the adverse health effects of weight cycling, obese persons who are unable to maintain reductions in weight may be eligible for surgery also.

## GASTRIC BYPASS AND VERTICAL BANDED GASTROPLASTY

The two most common surgeries for the treatment of obesity today are called gastric bypass and vertical banded gastroplasty. Both of these operations involve reversible alterations in the gastrointestinal tract that lead to early satiety (the feeling of fullness or gratification after eating).

In gastric bypass surgery, stomach size is reduced by the placement of staples across the upper portion of the stomach. In this procedure, food only enters this smaller section, called the pouch. The surgeon then attaches a section of the small intestine to an opening made in the pouch, which allows food to continue its normal passage through the digestive tract. Some surgeons believe that gastric bypass yields better weight control than vertical banded gastroplasty; however, it is also associated with more complications and, thus, a greater likelihood of reoperation to correct undesirable side effects.

**FIGURE 4-1.** *Gastric Bypass and Vertical Banded Gastroplasty*

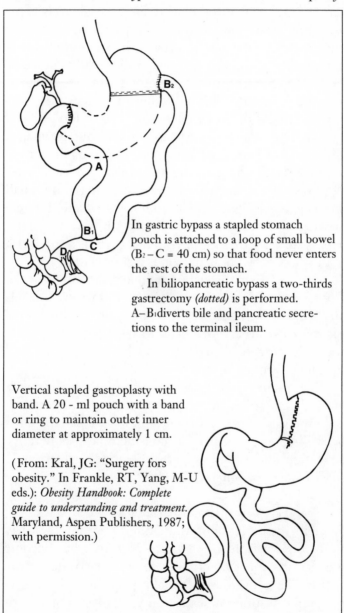

In gastric bypass a stapled stomach pouch is attached to a loop of small bowel ($B_2 - C$ = 40 cm) so that food never enters the rest of the stomach.

In biliopancreatic bypass a two-thirds gastrectomy *(dotted)* is performed. $A - B_1$ diverts bile and pancreatic secretions to the terminal ileum.

Vertical stapled gastroplasty with band. A 20 - ml pouch with a band or ring to maintain outlet inner diameter at approximately 1 cm.

(From: Kral, JG: "Surgery fors obesity." In Frankle, RT, Yang, M-U eds.): *Obesity Handbook: Complete guide to understanding and treatment.* Maryland, Aspen Publishers, 1987; with permission.)

Vertical banded gastroplasty is a simpler and more recent surgical development than gastric bypass. This technique also reduces stomach capacity by the use of staples but, unlike gastric bypass, the small intestine is not affected. Food passes through the small pouch created by the staples into the rest of the stomach, and then into the intestine. This procedure produces early satiety and limits the volume and the rate of food intake.

Neither of these operations is without problems. The pouches produced by stomach stapling are prone to gradual enlargement over a period of years and leakage around the staples or the area where the small intestine is attached can lead to serious infection. Some patients also develop stomach ulcers following gastric bypass surgery. In both operations, there is a small risk of death. A very obese person is a surgical risk.

Experience with vertical banded gastroplasty at the University of Iowa, where the procedure was developed, has shown that about 30 percent of patients receiving this surgery will drop to normal weight while about 80 percent of patients will have significant and sustained weight control.[7]

Successful surgical management of obesity requires more than a skilled and experienced surgeon rearranging the gastrointestinal tract. The obese patient must be willing to participate in considerable preoperative education and long-term postoperative evaluation. A strict feeding regimen must also be followed.

## LIPOSUCTION

Since its introduction in the United States in the early 1980s, liposuction (or suction lipectomy) has become the nation's most commonly requested cosmetic surgery.[8] The procedure is usually performed by a dermatological surgeon. Lipectomy involves the use of suction and a device called a cannula (a tube) to extract fat through small incisions in the skin. Some doctors and their patients consider suction lipectomy a viable treatment option for some types of obesity; however, others see it only as a "body contouring" procedure with no legitimate role in weight reduction.

Liposuction has been demonstrated to be relatively safe; between 1982 and 1990, eleven deaths were reported following more than 700,000 operations.[9] The procedure targets specific areas of fat accumulation, typically in the buttocks or thighs, for removal. Some physicians have advocated the use of liposuction to treat so-called female or gynecoid obesity, which primarily affects areas in the lower body. In this type of obesity, adipose tissue is highly localized; therefore, the application of liposuction can be considered appropriate. However, since liposuction can be expected to remove only 10 to 15 percent of the total adipose tissue, this procedure will not dramatically change the condition of an extremely obese individual.

Overall, there is significant controversy regarding the proper role of lipectomy in the treatment of obesity. Little long-term research has been carried out to determine if this type of surgical intervention is beneficial. Fat cells removed by liposuction may simply regenerate. If this is the case, liposuction may do more harm than good. Clearly, further study in this area is needed.

## DRUG TREATMENT OPTIONS

One area that has gained considerable attention in recent years is that of drug therapy for obesity. A great many appetite-suppressant drugs are sold over-the-counter and others are available through prescription.

These medications are currently recommended as short-term adjuncts to the treatment of obesity.

The use of appetite-suppressing drugs as a long-term therapy for obesity continues to be very controversial. Some medical doctors have gone on record supporting the use of such medications and testifying to their safety and effectiveness. Others have been reluctant to endorse the protracted use of appetite-suppressant drugs because of their unwanted side effects and because of data showing they are ineffective in achieving long-term weight loss.

A potentially serious side effect of some appetite-suppressant drugs is pulmonary hypertension, which can be life threatening. Other, milder, side effects include dry mouth, disrupted bowel habits, and insomnia. Studies indicate that, in addition, most obese patients regain weight after drug treatment ends. There is even some information to suggest that following drug therapy patients gain more weight than they lost during treatment, perhaps because they fail to adopt the lifestyle changes necessary to maintain proper body weight.

Nevertheless, proponents of drug therapy argue that expecting medications to guarantee permanent weight loss—in essence, to cure obesity—is both unrealistic and unfair. Other chronic health conditions—such as glaucoma, high blood pressure, and elevated cholesterol—are treated, but not cured, with long-term drug therapy. Such treatment is accepted as reasonable and in the best interest of the patient. Advocates of drug therapy ask, Why set higher standards for appetite-suppressing medications?

Critics of appetite-suppressants continue to point to the fact that these drugs are not proven safe, that deaths have been reported among patients taking such medications. For the time being, it appears that regulatory agencies like the federal Food and Drug Administration will continue to label these drugs as being for "short-term [a few weeks']" usage only.

Also of interest in the area of drug therapy is ongoing research into a pharmacological agent that specifically attacks fat cells—in effect, an obesity pill.[10] Such research is in the earliest stages, and the prospect of discovering a "magic bullet" for obesity anytime soon is unlikely. But there is hope that continued genetic research will one day make it possible to develop a drug that attacks fat without damaging normal tissue.

Each treatment option described in this chapter has unique advantages and disadvantages. While conservative treatment is attractive because it avoids surgery and keeps patients in charge of their own treatment, success rates remain stubbornly low. Some surgical procedures appear to have good success rates, but operations always entail considerable risk. Some individuals are not able or willing to take such chances. Drug therapy holds promise, but this, too, is not without risk and unwanted side effects; many doctors feel it is still basically experimental medicine. In all cases, the treatment of obesity is a long-term —perhaps lifelong—arrangement. Individuals are required to commit themselves to new lifestyles and new attitudes.

As one researcher noted in discussing the various options for reducing the prevalence of obesity, "Ultimately, prevention may have greater potential than does treatment."[11] The importance of preventive care is being recognized throughout the health care industry, and obesity appears to be one more area where prevention is the best medicine.

## APPENDIX ONE. *The Food Pyramid*
### *U.S.D.A. Recommended Number of Servings from the Six Food Groups*

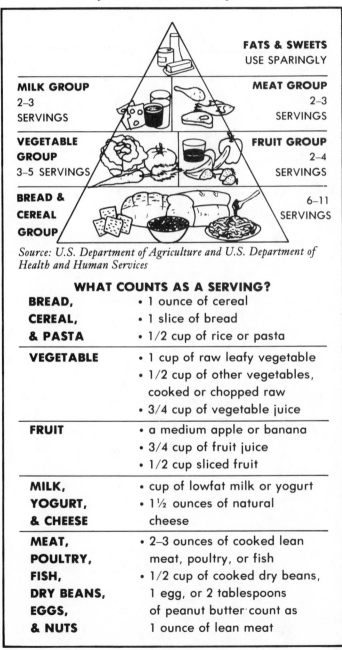

FATS & SWEETS
USE SPARINGLY

MILK GROUP
2–3
SERVINGS

MEAT GROUP
2–3
SERVINGS

VEGETABLE
GROUP
3–5 SERVINGS

FRUIT GROUP
2–4
SERVINGS

BREAD &
CEREAL
GROUP

6–11
SERVINGS

Source: U.S. Department of Agriculture and U.S. Department of Health and Human Services

## WHAT COUNTS AS A SERVING?

| | |
|---|---|
| **BREAD, CEREAL, & PASTA** | • 1 ounce of cereal<br>• 1 slice of bread<br>• 1/2 cup of rice or pasta |
| **VEGETABLE** | • 1 cup of raw leafy vegetable<br>• 1/2 cup of other vegetables, cooked or chopped raw<br>• 3/4 cup of vegetable juice |
| **FRUIT** | • a medium apple or banana<br>• 3/4 cup of fruit juice<br>• 1/2 cup sliced fruit |
| **MILK, YOGURT, & CHEESE** | • cup of lowfat milk or yogurt<br>• 1½ ounces of natural cheese |
| **MEAT, POULTRY, FISH, DRY BEANS, EGGS, & NUTS** | • 2–3 ounces of cooked lean meat, poultry, or fish<br>• 1/2 cup of cooked dry beans, 1 egg, or 2 tablespoons of peanut butter count as 1 ounce of lean meat |

**APPENDIX TWO.** *Overweight in America*
*National weight surveys are presented for people 20 to 74*
*years old. Figures represent percent of each group 20*
*percent or more over ideal weights.*

| | '80 | '91 | Increase from '80 to '91 |
|---|---|---|---|
| **Both sexes** | 25.4% | 33.3% | 31.1% |
| **Men** | 24.0 | 31.6 | 31.7 |
| **Women** | 26.5 | 35.0 | 32.1 |
| **White men** | 24.2 | 32.0 | 32.2 |
| **White women** | 24.4 | 33.5 | 37.3 |
| **Black men** | 25.7 | 31.5 | 22.6 |
| **Black women** | 44.3 | 49.6 | 12.0 |
| **Mexican–American men** | 31.0 | 39.5 | 27.4 |
| **Mexican–American women** | 41.4 | 47.9 | 15.7 |

| **By age group** | **20–34 years old** | **35–44** | **45–54** | **55–64** | **65–74** | **75 and over** |
|---|---|---|---|---|---|---|
| **Men** | 22.2% | 35.3% | 35.6% | 40.1% | 42.9% | 26.4% |
| **Women** | 25.1 | 36.9 | 41.6 | 48.5 | 39.8 | 30.9 |

All figures for women exclude pregnant women.

*Sources: Centers for Disease Control and Prevention, National Center for Health Statistics*

## APPENDIX THREE. *Higher Fat Foods*
*The American Heart Association recommends less than 30 percent total fat intake daily. Eat these foods once in a while or on special occasions.*

| 3-5 grams total fat | Serving Size | Metric Measure | Calories | Total Fat g |
|---|---|---|---|---|
| Milk, 2% fat | 8 fl oz | 240 ml | 121 | 5 |
| Buttermilk, 2% fat | 8 fl oz | 240 ml | 112 | 5 |
| Part-skim mozzarella cheese | 1 oz | 30 g | 79 | 5 |
| Cream cheese, light | 1 oz | 30 g | 62 | 5 |
| Cottage cheese, creamed | ½ cup | 110 g | 117 | 5 |
| Chicken soup with noodles | 1 cup | 241 g | 82 | 3 |
| Beef and vegetable soup | 1 cup | 240 g | 83 | 3 |
| Chocolate chip cookie | 1 oz | 30 g | 139 | 4 |
| **6-10 grams total fat** | | | | |
| Whole milk | 8 fl oz | 240 ml | 150 | 8 |
| Yogurt, plain whole milk | 1 cup | 225 g | 138 | 7 |
| Yogurt, flavored whole milk | 1 cup | 225 g | 268 | 7 |
| American cheese | 1 oz | 30 g | 106 | 9 |
| Cheddar cheese | 1 oz | 30 g | 114 | 9 |
| Ice cream | ½ cup | 68 g | 135 | 7 |
| Ice cream cone | 1 | — | 157 | 7 |
| Bacon | 2 slices | 12 g | 73 | 6 |
| Spaghetti with meat sauce | 1 cup | 250 g | 239 | 10 |
| New England clam chowder | 1 cup | 248 g | 163 | 7 |
| Plain hamburger | 1 | 90 g | 274 | 10 |
| Frankfurter, chicken | 1½ oz | 42 g | 110 | 8 |
| Bologna | 1 oz | 28 g | 90 | 8 |
| Brownie | 1 large | 40 g | 172 | 9 |
| Sugar cookie | 1 oz | 30 g | 137 | 8 |
| Biscuit | 2 oz | 55 g | 165 | 7 |
| Potato chips | 1 oz | 30 g | 156 | 10 |
| Popcorn, microwave popped | 3 cups | 30 g | 118 | 6 |
| Oatmeal cookie | 1 oz | 30 g | 126 | 6 |
| Blueberry or bran muffin | 1 large | 55 g | 161 | 6 |
| Pancakes, 4″ diameter | 5 | 110 g | 388 | 7 |

| 11-15 grams total fat | Serving Size | Metric Measure | Calories | Total Fat g |
|---|---|---|---|---|
| Ice cream bar (½ cup) | 3 oz | 84 g | 178 | 13 |
| Taco | 1 | — | 245 | 15 |
| Fajita, steak | 1 | — | 224 | 11 |
| Enchilada | 1 | — | 229 | 13 |
| Pork sausage | 3 links | — | 144 | 12 |
| Frankfurter, beef and pork | 1½ oz | 42 g | 136 | 12 |
| Beef stew | 1 cup | 245 g | 303 | 14 |
| English muffin sandwich with egg, cheese, Canadian bacon | 1 | — | 297 | 13 |
| Fried chicken (breast) | 3 oz | 84 g | 255 | 15 |
| Cheese pizza, 6" diameter | 1 | — | 422 | 13 |
| Cheeseburger, single patty | 1 | — | 326 | 14 |
| Chili with beans | 1 cup | 255 g | 272 | 11 |
| Butter | 1 tbsp | 15 g | 102 | 12 |
| Italian dressing | 2 tbsp | 30 g | 138 | 14 |
| Mayonnaise | 1 tbsp | 15 g | 99 | 11 |
| Croissant | 1 | 55 g | 172 | 12 |
| Hot dog with bun | 1 | 98 g | 264 | 15 |
| Peanut butter | 2 tbsp | 30 g | 176 | 15 |
| French fries | 16 medium | 70 g | 210 | 13 |
| Doughnut, raised, glazed | 1 small | 55 g | 233 | 14 |

### 16-20 grams total fat

| | Serving Size | Metric Measure | Calories | Total Fat g |
|---|---|---|---|---|
| Macaroni and cheese | 1 cup | — | 399 | 18 |
| Lasagna, 3" × 3" | 1 cup | — | 383 | 19 |
| Sandwich, breaded fish | 1 | 158 g | 424 | 19 |
| Peanuts, roasted | ¼ cup | 40 g | 232 | 20 |
| Chocolate cake | 2" wedge | 75 g | 447 | 19 |
| Blue cheese dressing | 2 tbsp | 30 g | 154 | 16 |

### 21-26 grams total fat

| | Serving Size | Metric Measure | Calories | Total Fat g |
|---|---|---|---|---|
| Burrito | 1 | — | 499 | 23 |
| Club sandwich | 1 | — | 483 | 22 |
| Pepperoni pizza, 6" diameter | 1 | — | 653 | 25 |
| Tuna salad | ½ cup | 103 g | 279 | 24 |
| Polish sausage | 3 oz | 84 g | 277 | 24 |
| Spare ribs | 3 oz | 84 g | 310 | 26 |

# SOURCE NOTES

## INTRODUCTION

I-1. University of California at Berkeley Wellness Letter 10(5):2, 1994.

I-2. Bray GA: Barriers to the treatment of obesity. (Editorial.) *Annals of Internal Medicine* 115:152, 1991.

## CHAPTER ONE

1-1. Hearings Before the Subcommittee on Regulation, Business Opportunities, and Energy of the House Committee on Small Business. March 26, 1990.

1-2. Canning H, Mayer J: Obesity—its possible effect on college acceptance. *New England Journal of Medicine* 275:1172, 1966.

1-3. Taitz Leonard L: *The Obese Child.* Blackwell Scientific Publications, 1983.

1-4. Forman MR, Trowbridge FL, Gentry EM, et al: Overweight adults in the United States. *American Journal of Clinical Nutrition* 44:410, 1986.

1-5. Colditz GS: Economic costs of obesity. *American Journal of Clinical Nutrition* 55:503S, 1992.

1-6. U.S. Department of Health and Human Services Public Health Service: *Healthy People 2000: National Health Promotion and Disease Prevention Objectives.* 1991

1-7. Doherty C, Mason E: Clinically severe obesity: A review. *Iowa Medicine* 82:335, 1992.

## CHAPTER TWO

2–1. Danforth E, Sims EAH: Obesity and efforts to lose weight. (Editorial.) *New England Journal of Medicine* 327:1947, 1992.

2–2. Braitman LE, Adlin V, Stanton JL: Obesity and caloric intake. *Journal of Chronic Diseases* 38: 727, 1985.

2–3. Romieu I, Willet WC, Stampfer MJ, et al: Energy intake and other determinants of relative weight. *American Journal of Clinical Nutrition* 47:406, 1988.

2–4. Lichtman SW, Pisarska K, Berman ER, et al: Discrepancy between self-reported and actual caloric intake and exercise in obese patients. *New England Journal of Medicine* 327:1893, 1992.

2–5. Iowa Department of Agriculture and Land Stewardship: *It's a whole new world.* 1991.

2–6. U.S Department of Health and Human Services Public Health Service: *Healthy People 2000: National Health Promotion and Disease Prevention Objectives.* 1991

2–7. Bouchard C: Current understanding of the etiology of obesity: Genetic and nongenetic factors. *American Journal of Clinical Nutrition* 53:1561S, 1991.

2–8. Bouchard C: Current understanding of the etiology of obesity: Genetic and nongenetic factors. *American Journal of Clinical Nutrition* 53:1561S, 1991.

2–9. Howard BV, Bogardus C, Ravussin E, et al: Studies of the etiology of obesity in Pima Indians. *American Journal of Clinical Nutrition* 53:1577S, 1991.

2–10. Pettitt DJ, Knowler WC: Diabetes and obesity in the Pima Indians: A cross-generational vicious cycle. *Journal of Obesity and Weight Regulation* 7:61, 1988.

2–11. Burke GL, Savage PJ, Manolio TA, et al: Correlates of obesity in young black and white women: The CARDIA study. *American Journal of Public Health* 82:1621, 1992.

2–12. Burros M: Eating well. *The New York Times* March 4, 1992.

2–13. Patterson BH, Block G: Food choices and the cancer guidelines. *American Journal of Public Health* 78:282, 1988.

2–14. Bennet EM: Weight loss practices of overweight adults. *American Journal of Clinical Nutrition* 53:1519S, 1991.

2–15. Dietz WH, Gortmaker SL: Do we fatten our children at the television set? Obesity and television viewing in children and adolescents. *Pediatrics* 75:807, 1985.

2–16. Dietz WH, Gortmaker SL: Factors within the physical environment associated with childhood obesity. *American Journal of Clinical Nutrition* 39:619, 1984.

2–17. O'Neil PM, Jarrel MP: Psychological aspects of obesity and very-low-calorie diets. *American Journal of Clinical Nutrition* 56:185S, 1992.

2–18. Wadden TA, Stunkard AJ: Social and psychological consequences of obesity. *Annals of Internal Medicine* 103:1062, 1985.

2–19. Leon GR, Roth L: Obesity: Psychological causes, correlations, and speculations. *Psychological Bulletin* 84:117, 1977.

2–20. O'Neil PM, Jarrel MP: Psychological aspects of obesity and very-low-calorie diets. *American Journal of Clinical Nutrition* 56:185S, 1992.

2–21. O'Neil PM, Jarrel MP: Psychological aspects of obesity and very-low-calorie diets. *American Journal of Clinical Nutrition* 56:185S, 1992.

2–22. Taitz L: *The Obese Child.* Blackwell Scientific Publications, 1983.

## CHAPTER THREE

3–1. Rabkin SW, Mathewson FA, Hsu PH: Relation of bodyweight to development of ischemic heart disease in a cohort of young North American men after a 26-year observation period. The Manitoba Study. *American Journal of Cardiology* 39:452, 1977.

3–2. Sorlie P, Gordon T, Kannel WB: Body build and mortality: The Framingham Study. *Journal of the American Medical Association* 243:1828, 1980.

3–3. American Heart Association: *Heart and Stroke Facts 1994.*

3–4. Hubert HB, Feinleib M, McNamara PM, Castelli WP: Obesity as an independent risk factor for cardiovascular disease: A 26-year follow-up of participants in the Framingham Heart Study. *Circulation* 67:968, 1983.

3–5. *Mayo Clinic Family Health Book* (Larson DE, editor). New York: William Morrow and Co., Inc., 1990.

3–6. Tannenbaum A: Relationship of body weight to cancer incidence. *Archives of Pathology* 30:509, 1940.

3–7. The Work Study Group on Diet, Nutrition, and Cancer: American Cancer Society Guidelines on Diet, Nutrition, and Cancer. *CA* 41:334, 1991.

3–8. The Work Study Group on Diet, Nutrition, and Cancer: American Cancer Society Guidelines on Diet, Nutrition, and Cancer. *CA* 41:334, 1991.

3–9. Friedl KE, Plymate SR: Effect of obesity on reproduction in the female. *Journal of Obesity and Weight Regulation* 4:129, 1985.

3–10. O'Neil PM, Jarrel MP: Psychological aspects of

obesity and very-low-calorie diets. *American Journal of Clinical Nutrition* 56:185S, 1992.

3–11. Stunkard A, Mendelson M: Disturbances in body image of some obese persons. *Journal of the American Dietetic Association* 38:328, 1961.

3–12. Lissner L, Odell PM, D'Agnostino RB, et al: Variability of body weight and health outcomes in the Framingham population. *New England Journal of Medicine* 324:1839, 1991.

## CHAPTER FOUR

4–1. University of California at Berkeley Wellness Letter 105:2, 1994.

4–2. Hirsch J: Barriers to treating obesity. (Letter.) *Annals of Internal Medicine* 115:656, 1991.

4–3. Bray G: In: *Health and Obesity* by Peter T. Kuo. Raven, 1983.

4–4. Wadden TA, Stunkard AJ, Brownell KD: Very low calorie diets: Their efficacy, safety and future. *Annals of Internal Medicine* 99:675, 1983.

4–5. Pi-Sunyer FX: The role of very low calorie diets in obesity. *American Journal of Clinical Nutrition* 56:240S, 1992.

4–6. Special Medical Reports: NIH consensus statement covers treatment of obesity. *American Family Practitioner* 44:305, 1991.

4–7. Mason EE, et al: Ten years of vertical banded gastroplasty for severe obesity. *Problems in General Surgery* 9:280, 1992.

4–8. Mladick RA, Morrel RL: Sixteen months experince with the Illouz technique of lipolysis. *Annals of Plastic Surgery* 16:220, 1986.

4–9. Fredricks S, Anastasi GW, Baker JL, et al: Complications and deaths from lipoplasty. In: Ad Hoc

Committee on New Procedures. Five-year updated evaluation of the American Society of Plastic and Reconstructive Surgeons. ASPRS, 1987.

4–10. Godwin FK: From the Alcohol, Drug Abuse, and Mental Health Administration (news article). *Journal of the American Medical Association* 267:910, 1992.

4–11. Bennet EM: Weight loss practices of overweight adults. *American Journal of Clinical Nutrition* 53:1519S, 1991.

# FOR FURTHER READING

Cassell, Dana K. *Encyclopedia of Obesity & Eating Disorders*. New York: Facts on File, 1993.

Landau, Elaine. *Weight: A Teenage Concern*. New York: Dutton Children's Books, 1991.

Lee, Sally. *New Theories on Diet and Nutrition*. New York: Franklin Watts, 1990.

Silverstein, Alvin, et al. *So You Think You're Fat?* New York: HarperCollins Children's Books, 1991.

Sonder, Ben. *Eating Disorders: When Food Turns Against You*. New York: Franklin Watts, 1993.

Storlie, Jean and Henry A. Jordan, eds. *Evaluation and Treatment of Obesity*. Champaign, Ill.: Human Kinetics Publications, 1988.

Taitz, Leonard. *The Obese Child*. London: Blackwell Scientific Publications, 1983.

# INDEX

Abdominal fat, 25, 26, 38
Activity levels, 19, 26–27, 28, 33–37
   exercise and, 36–37, 62, 63
   technology and, 34–36
Adipose tissue. *See* Fat
Adult-onset obesity, 28
African Americans, 38–39
Age:
   body fat content and, 19–20
   at onset of obesity, 26–28
Anti-cellulite creams, 14
Anxiety, 36, 41, 42, 55
Appetite-regulation disorders, 28, 33
Appetite-suppressant drugs, 73–75
Arthritis, 52

Atherosclerosis, 46–47
Attitudinal factors, 39, 63

Behavioral factors, 39
Behavioral modification, 61–66, 68
Binge eating, 42
Body fat. *See* Fat
Body image, 54–55
Body Mass Index (BMI), 20–21, 24
Body types, attractiveness and, 14–15
Bulimia, 42

Calipers, 20, 25
Cancer, 9, 10, 36, 49–52
Cardiovascular disease, 9, 21, 46–47
Causes of obesity, 31–43
   environmental factors, 39–41
   ethnicity, 38–39

# ABOUT THE AUTHOR

Daniel McMillan, a graduate of the University of Iowa School of Journalism and Mass Communication, is currently a medical editor at the University of Iowa College of Medicine. Mr. McMillan's most recent book for Franklin Watts is *Winning the Battle Against Drugs: Rehabilitation Programs*.

Mr. McMillan lives in Iowa City, Iowa, and enjoys travel, camping, and long walks with his dog, Georgia.